# THE DEPRESSION CURE

I0464568

## HOW TO OVERCOME DEPRESSION AND BECOME DEPRESSION FREE

By Patricia A Carlisle

# Introduction

I want to thank you and congratulate you for choosing the book, *"THE DEPRESSION CURE: How to overcome depression and become depression free"*.

This book contains proven steps and strategies on how to overcome depression and become depression free.

More people are feeling a wide range of symptoms of depression. Everyone experience the normal ups and downs of life, and everyone feels sad or has "the blues" sometimes. But if helplessness and hopelessness won't go away don't worry.

The good news is no matter how hopeless you feel, here are some things you can do to feel better. Remember the most severe depression is treatable. So, if your depression is keeping you from living the life you want to, don't hesitate to download this book.

**Here is what you will learn:**

- *HOW TO TACKLE DEPRESSION HEAD-ON THE RIGHT WAY*

- *SYMPTOMS AND SIGNS OF DEPRESSION*

- *TYPES OF DEPRESSION*

- *HOW IT MANIFEST IN PEOPLE*

- *TREATMENT OF DEPRESSION*

- *THERAPY/MEDICATION*

- *HOW TO LIVE WITH DEPRESSION*

- *HOW TO CHANGE YOUR DIET AND LIFESTYLE*

Thanks again for choosing this book, I hope you enjoy it!

# TABLE OF CONTENT

# Chapter 1

faces - moods

## MOOD DISORDER IS DEPRESSION
### Tackling depression head-on the right way

Recovery begins when we overcome depression and become totally depression free. Treatment for depression began when one analyzes the causes, and learns the symptoms of depression. Depression cure needs much patience from both the patient and the physician. Depression unlike sadness and happiness is not a normal human emotion. Naturally, many people do not realize they are depressed, and let this ailment go unnoticed.

However, it is because there is every possibility for this serious mood disorder to cause disruption to normal social life, and even death one needs to look at the signs.

When you feel lonely, and down in the dumps, you take a walk or a refreshing drink and you feel bright and cheerful once again. And those situations when you feel that your thoughts and feelings, your since of well being seem to have disappeared, gone on a vacation, you have to sit up and straighten your tie. Depression cure, unlike relief from stress does not happen naturally.

In most cases, you will be advised to begin treatment as soon as you detect the first signs and symptoms of depression. You do not have many methods to diagnose mood swings and depressive state of mind, your physician will not be able to help you with your element unless you come forward and discuss the symptoms with him or her.

# Chapter 2

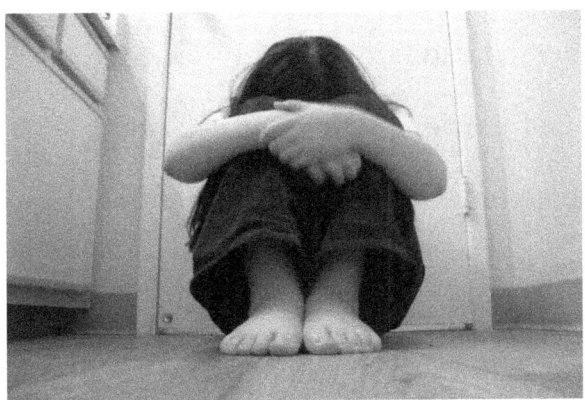

## SYMPTOMS AND SIGNS OF DEPRESSION

### 1. Metabolic changes

**a. Significant changes in appetite levels:**

Appetite changes – those with typical symptoms show loss of appetite while those with atypical symptoms will show an increase in appetite. Also, a very significant weight loss or weight gain could manifest in depressed individuals.

**b. Changes in sleep pattern:** Insomnia, fatigue and pain – these are the first symptoms of the impact of depression, and physical and health. Early waking in the morning adds to restlessness. In addition you may develop cramps and problems with your digestion system which sometimes accompany the signs and symptoms for depression.

2. **Mental changes:**

   a. **Feelings of pessimism, irrational guilt or hopelessness:** A person suffering from depression will go through emotions ranging from helplessness to negative thinking about the present and the future. They remain obsessed by feelings of guilt that seem to develop from nowhere. To overcome depression, depression cure will focus on keeping the mood and feelings of the individual stable.

   b. **Continuous sad feeling:** The dominant feeling for people who experience depression will be one of sadness. It is the lack of positive emotions which is caused by the way the chemicals in the brain reacts. Often, people in a depressed state will slip back in a sad state even if you try to cheer up them up.

c. **Irritation at the slightest aggravation:**

Lack of sleep combined with poor energy levels due to disruptions in the metabolic activity contribute to a very sensitive mental state. Any changes around the person will cause him or her to explode, and behave in an irrational manner. If this symptom is present, then depression cure is tuff, if the person will have enormous trouble getting ready to overcoming depression.

3. **Orientation and energy:**

a. **Significant decrease in energy levels:**

Altered brain structure during depression leads to less efficient working of your metabolism. The body does not have sufficient energy to carry out routine metabolic activities. Good energy levels are required to overcome depression. We will read about eating well, later on in this book, to sustain energy levels, since this is essential for developing a cure for your depression.

b. **Having difficulty remembering things:**

Brain activity remains superficial, and the person does not relate to their present activities. He or she will lose interest in day-to-day activities. Lack of concentration by the brain leads to memory lapses and disorientation. First step to become depression free is to take steps to develop a steady thought process. When her or she is able to think straight without becoming distracted, then they will be ready to overcome depression, and on your way to becoming depression free. One way to do this is to write your thoughts down, for example, keeping a diary. In the beginning, you will find you will not be able to control the direction of your thoughts.

But over time, you will discover a definite trend to your thought process.

c. **Significantly distanced social pattern:**
Persons with depression will have trouble remembering details. Subsequently they will have problems making decisions, and connecting with social circles meaningfully. Depressive moods that have no real basis will make the person stop his or her task without really completing the job. For instance, the sight of flowers may cause a negative response to people who are depressed after experiencing a tragic event like a death in the family. Getting help from friends and relatives is a good way to overcome depression. Good social contact is a natural depression cure mechanism.

# Chapter 3

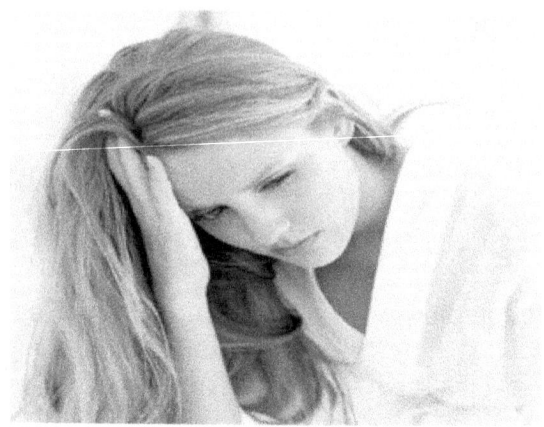

## TYPES OF DEPRESSION

Knowing what type of depression you are experiencing is essential in choosing an effective depression cure treatment plan. Depression can manifest as mood disorders, and overwhelming mood swings which eventually can prevent a person from completing their treatment plan. If you are feeling lifeless, empty, or in an uninterested mental states, and don't know what type of depression you may have, here is a list of a few depression types you can talk over with your doctor.

1) **Situational Depression:** Any life-altering event such as losing your job, death of someone you love can

trigger depression. Stress response syndrome happens when the person faces an unusual situation in life. Symptoms of situational depression include long periods of sadness, nervousness, or worries about unrelated things in your life that disturb you. In most cases, situational depression will disappear with time, but sometimes medical intervention may be required to overcome depression. Your depression will heal naturally in most cases.

2) **Major Depression:** Major depression impacts 7.32% of most people in the Country. True to its character, Major Depression is very debilitating; it disrupts the normal functioning of a depressed person. In this type, it is difficult to overcome depression and have complete depression cure. Other symptoms are changes in sleep and eating patterns, interference during decision making or thinking, irritability, physical pain and guilt feelings are the most commonly manifested symptoms. More than 6% of Americans have undergone Major

Depression. Over 75% of the patients with this mood disorder overcome depression when treated with medicines and talk therapy. This type has a 90% depression cure rate.

3) **Bipolar Disorder**: Manic Depressive Disorder is another name for Bipolar Disorder. With this disorder, it will be difficult to overcome depression and have complete depression cure. To recognize this symptoms in depressive disorder, recognize some of the mood swings in the person such as, racing thoughts, high energy, poor judgment and excitement. Even though Bipolar Disorder only affects about 3% of the population, due to the severity of the symptoms immediate and effective steps must start immediately to overcome depression. You will also find a lower rate for a cure for depression, and a higher incidence of suicide in this type of depression than in others.

The subtypes of Bipolar Disorder are:

    a. Bipolar I

b. Bipolar II

c. Cyclothymic disorder

d. Other related bipolar disorders

Treatment is affected through the use of a class of medications known as mood stabilizers.

**4)** **Psychotic Depression:** Delusions – false beliefs and hallucinations – imaginary sights and noises pre-dominate this depressive disorder. In psychotic depression, individuals become very reluctant to leave their beds, and sometimes do not even speak. In effect, these depressed individuals lose touch with reality. To overcome depression, and have complete depression cure, there are two kinds of medications; one is a medication that's for treating psychosis, and two, a medication for treating depression. Also the rate of getting cured from these medications is significantly lower due to the complex nature of mood disorder.

**5) Premenstrual Dysphoric Disorder** (PMDD): Hormonal changes occur in women during their premenstrual stage in life.  Premenstrual Dysphoric Disorder, is a grave disorder characterized by the following symptoms:

    i.  Anxiety

    ii.  Fatigue

    iii.  Overwhelming emotional surges

    iv.  High level of irritability

    v.  Concentration problems

    vi.  Wide fluctuation in sleep and eating habits

    vii.  Major mood swings

This type of depression upsets the thoughts and behavior and the women become very moody.  You can expect PMDD to onset during second-half of that person's menstrual cycle.  For most women, depression heals quickly.  The mood disorder upsets normal functioning, and thereby disrupts or alters relationships.  Over 82.4% of women face this once every 30 days, but they overcome naturally.  Check with your doctor and ask for nutritional supplements, and medicines to help you through the dark phase to overcome depression.

6) **Atypical Depression**: The most dominant symptom of Atypical Depression would be lethargy in the limbs. Individuals having Atypical Depression would overeat, and in most cases oversleep which is not a typical symptom for depression – hence the name. Individuals with Atypical Depression can have trouble with relationships, gain weight, and be irritable most of the time. Since the symptoms are not so overwhelming, these signs and symptoms escape their notice. Learn to recognize the signs and symptoms first, and then you can begin your depression cure treatment, usually with medicines to overcome depression.

7) **Persistent Depressive Disorder**: Just as the name indicates, Persistent Depressive Disorder last for long durations, sometimes for years. Another name for persistent depressive disorder is dysthymia. Typical

symptoms would be loss of esteem, changes in appetite patterns, and energy deprivation along with disruptions in sleep patterns. Individuals with Persistent Depressive Disorder will have feelings of hopelessness, and trouble in decision-making situations. People with this type of mood disorder have trouble overcoming depression. According to one study, at least 2.52% of Americans have suffered from this mood disorder. Best treatment options available for relief of depression are Talk Therapy and medication, either alone, or in combination for an effective treatment for this type of depression.

8) **Seasonal Affective Disorder** (SAD): Seasonal Affective Disorder occurs in individuals during the extreme winter months. Weight gain, daytime fatigue, escalating irritability, and feelings of anxiety are the symptoms of this mental health condition. For most mood disorder individuals, Light therapy can effectively

restore your mood, and overcome depression. and result in a full depression cure.

9) **Postpartum Depression:** Once woman gives birth to her child; significant changes in her hormone levels take place. This can develop feelings of hopelessness and inadequacy in them. This happens in about 90% of all women, and in about 20% the depression can be serious enough to warrant treatment. Talk therapy along with medication can effectively help overcome depression and treat this mood disorder.

# Chapter 4

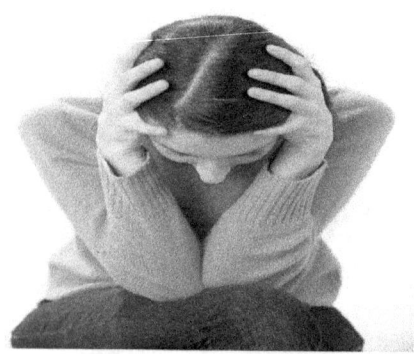

## CAUSES FOR DEPRESSION

During depression, the person has less control over his or her emotions. Causes may be physical or mental, and in some cases even social. Let us examine some of the depression causing factors that will help use to avoid depressive situations.

1. **Careers with high incidence of depression causing factors:** Pilots and actors due to their high commitments, politicians, and stuntmen who perform for circus acts come down with severe depression. High

tensions of their job combined with inadequate recognition creates mood disorders.

2. **Substance abuse:** People who use drugs may exhibit mood swings if they have and addiction. You must first overcome any addiction before you can work on overcoming depression.

3. **Medical illness or medication associated with treatment:** Lyme disease, Addison's disease, medication such as interferon, circadian rhythm, and sleep apnea.

4. **Death, lifestyle changing event:** Sudden changes in lifestyle such as losing a job or spouse, or experiencing death or destruction can bring emotional trauma, and make the person depressed.

5. **Genetics:** People who have family members who exhibited depression will most likely contract this illness at some point in their lives. Most illnesses have well researched solutions to overcome depression.

6. **Personal problems:** Facing very difficult social or financial situations can cause mood disorders.

7. **Borderline Personality Disorder:** This medical condition can bring about extreme states of depression. Psychological reaction to mood disturbance manifests as borderline personality disorder in individuals having identity problems. This type is difficult to diagnose, but many people overcome the depression that develops.

# Chapter 5

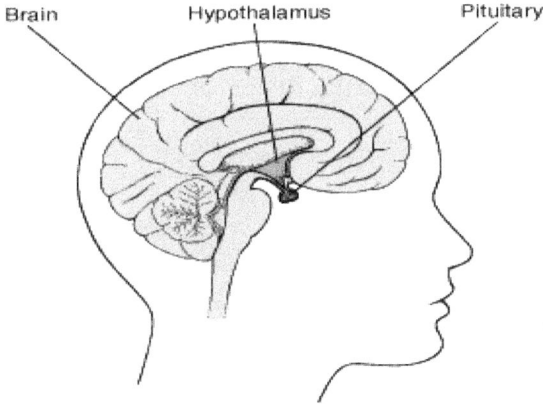

Brain      Hypothalamus      Pituitary

## HOW DEPRESSION MANIFEST IN PEOPLE

The chance to develop depression is higher in women than in men. Biological life cycle in women combines with hormonal imbalances brought on socio-psychological factors such as onset of menstruation, or the birth of a child. These unique events in the life of women isolate them from man bringing on the feelings of helplessness and rejection too frequently.

However, they can easily overcome depression. New responsibilities or sudden changes in lifestyle can upset the hormonal balance. Hormones maintain the well being of the person by regulating the metabolism. Through chemical in your body, they interlink to make a messaging system. One frequently finds hormones out of balance during the menopause phase, or the first menstrual occurrence for women.

Hormones are responsible for moods and emotions in the person. The "feel-good" chemical neurotransmitters in the human body such as serotonin or dopamine become less, because the metabolism is coping with some other change such as involving in milk production, or instigating the menstrual cycle...leading to depression.

Severe cases of Premenstrual syndrome may occur during changes that occur before menstruation begins and ovulation occurs. This premenstrual syndrome is called premenstrual dysphoric disorder (PMDD).

1) **Depression in men and older adults.** Older adults do not show extreme signs of depression or grief. Complicated long lasting grief like caregiver after the passing of loved one, or failure in some point in life versus

the actual state of depression may not be so obvious. Generally, you will not find older adults exhibiting signs of grief, and it is likely that one might miss the obvious signs of depression when it occurs. Complicated long lasting grief requires treatment just as major depression does. It takes time to overcome and get relief from depression.

2) **Teen depression instances.** Other than the normal list of symptoms associated with depression, signs and symptoms associated with teen depressions involve feelings and emotional mood disorders that come with reaching puberty. Since most of their emotions are not channelized, the reaction of teens to different social peer will be unbalanced. Depression could result from not achieving the normal things they see other older individuals achieve, and from the passing of a close relative or exposure to a violent incident.

We should first learn to recognize the symptoms of depression as well as the causes. Effective mood disorder therapy for teens begins by knowing what caused it. Depression in teens may result from one or more of the following conditions:

a) Physical or emotional abuse
b) Heredity
c) Social achievement pressure
d) Low confidence levels
e) Financial hardships
f) Parents are divorced or divorcing
g) Romantic entanglement
h) Academic pressures
i) "Become an adult" pressure

All growing children will feel pressure when they are exposed to society, and many will be unsure how to react. Being unaware of what goes on in the world, most of them will experience defeat at every turn. This can form depression among teens. Moreover, everyone may not be rich, or have enough talent to score high marks in their academics. One can introduce counseling in school to help children cope with social pressures, and help them overcome any emotional setbacks.

## DEPRESSION AND SUICIDE

Some depression can lead to suicide. Every situation may seem hopeless for people undergoing mood disorder. Many people have overcome depression with treatment and support. Here are some signs that will help you to recognize signs of suicide:

- Person talks about being trapped.

- Exhibits signs of hopelessness.
- Direct talks about suicide or indirect references to death and dying.
- Makes 'goodbye visits' to friends and relatives.
- Shows sudden calmness during depressive state.

- Behaves extremely recklessly like over speeding, or walking on parapets of high rise buildings.

# Chapter 6

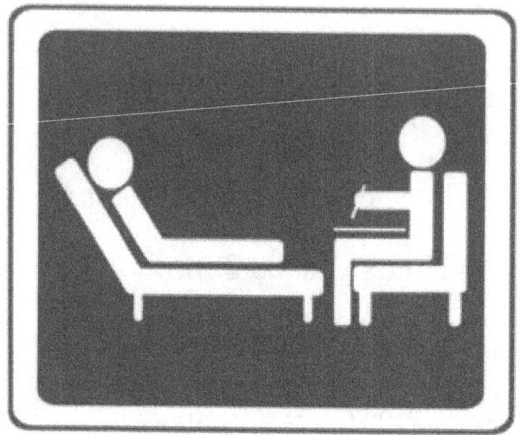

## TREATMENTS FOR DEPRESSION

In most cases, there is rearrangement of nerve cells in the brain when a person suffers from depression. Sometimes, as in the case of *Seasonal Affective Disorder*, substituting or rearranging the cause for the mood disturbance will restore the person to his or her original state of mind. Medication is required to help promote communication between nerve cells. One could also use talk therapy or light therapy to treat depression.

## OTHER THERAPY

### EMDR Therapy/Exposure Therapy

These types of therapy for anxiety disorder treatment consists of getting the individual to face their fears by exposing the individual to the very same objects that seem to trigger their anxiety. This situation is design to be harmless, and only helps the patient learn to overcome his or her anxiety in a gradual manner.

Most Psychotherapy usually takes years to show results. In EMDR, disturbing effects of emotional imbalance can be erased within a week or two. Distressing memories bring about mood disturbances necessitating psychotherapy treatment. Eye-movement Desensitization and Reprocessing (EMDR) utilizes external stimuli mainly movements of eye laterally, and may also use audio stimulation, or tapping with the hand.

EMDR finds use in improved symptoms associated with posttraumatic stress disorder (PTSD). Procedure entails an eight stage treatment method, but it's possible to overcome depression and have complete depression cure. Metabolic mechanisms that normally cope with situational disturbances are overwhelmed when exposed to distressing traumatic experiences necessitating the need for EMDR. The effectiveness of EMDR was reported to be the same as when using SSRI or exposure therapy.

## Vagus Nerve Stimulation (VNS)

Vagus Nerve Stimulation for mood disorder patients operates by sending electrical signal through to the mood controlling regions of the brain through the vagus nerve present in the neck region. Passing these electronic pulses stimulate chemical action that elevates the mood of the person. One may not overcome depression since the results vary from person to person.

## Transcranial Magnetic Stimulation (TMS)

Most severe depressive disorder individuals can be cured with repetitive Transcranial magnetic stimulation (rTMS). These people low levels in life are due to a low mood and serious repeated attacks of depression. In rTMS, one witnesses electrical impulses being sent to a portion inside the skull where moods originate. rTMS does not seem to have any side effects like causing seizures.

## Talk Therapy For Depression

Suitable for mild to moderate depression, you may utilize talk therapy in various forms. *Cognitive Behavioral Therapy* (CBT) improves behavior and related thought patterns, and thereby avoids links to depression. This will help you completely overcome depression. One can develop a realistic viewpoint of the ways your mood changes with your relationships in *Interpersonal Therapy* (IPT). Unconscious sublimely feelings or unresolved issues can contribute to mood or behavior. You understand this from *Psychodynamic Psychotherapy* (PP). When treatment in traditional manner using medication and talk therapy does not provide the required results one may have to adopt *Brain Stimulation*

*Therapies* (BST). One such therapy is *Electroconvulsive*

*Therapy* (ECT). In this, repeated shocks helps you overcome

your depression and sometimes a total cure.

# Chapter 7

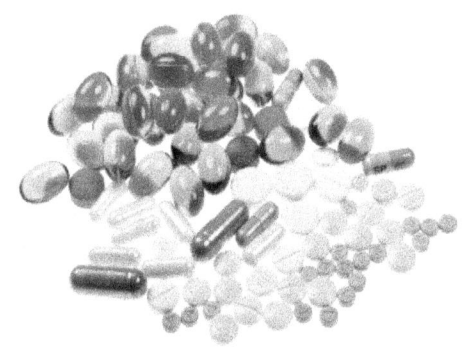

## MEDICATION

Chemicals present in the brain used for conveying information between nerve cells are called neurotransmitters. Norepinephrine, serotonin, and dopamine are the neurotransmitters targeted by medicine prescribed for depression. To feel a good thought and feeling, and a positive sense of well being depend on the hormone balance in our body at a particular time. Our metabolism controls the balance through neurotransmitters, and controls are feelings of being happy or sad.

Antidepressants have evolved over time with the latest versions termed as Norepinephrine Reuptake Inhibitors (SNRI), and Selective Serotonin Reuptake Inhibitors (SSRI). Fluoxetine (Prozac), Sertraline (Zoloft), Paroxetine (Paxil), and Escitalopram (Lexapro) are examples of SSRIs prescribed for depression. Duloxetine (Cymbalta), and venlafaxine (Effexor) are commonly prescribed SNRIs. Common side effects are seen when the patient fist begins to take these medicines. For example, shakes, insomnia and nausea along with headaches are the command symptoms one sees.

Older generation of antidepressant medication includes Monoamine oxidase inhibitors (MAOI), and Tricyclics. The first antidepressant medicines were MAOIs. They have a very good affect in helping you overcome your depression. But the side effects prohibit their use. You may find them working well for those who have too much sleep, or experiencing an increase in appetite. However, when taken in combination with certain other medicines like allergy or cold medication, herbal supplements, prescription pain relievers, or birth control pills they can cause a fatal increase in blood pressure. Other side effects many individuals experience when taking SSRI and MAOI together are confusion, stiffness of the muscle, hearth rhythm, and blood pressure changes seizures, sweating, and hallucinations. Many of the conditions may be life threatening. At the time the doctor issues the prescription for theses medicines, be sure to ask for a list of foods and medication to avoid.

Tricyclics followed MAOI. These antidepressant medications are powerful, but like MAOIs have their own side effects. Tricyclics such as nortriptyline are used commonly, but may cause dizziness in older people. If overdosed they could prove dangerous. Other side effects include dry mouth, drowsiness, and in most instances weight gain.

Medication takes full effect only after a month or more. After this period, the individual may feel better, but must carry on with the medication until the doctor tell you to stop. If you feel you no longer need the medication, discuss it with your doctor because if you suddenly stop taking your medication this could result in development of withdrawal symptoms resulting in a relapse. Individuals exhibiting recurrent signs of depression when taken off the medication will be asked to continue the medicines indefinitely to overcome depression and have complete depression cure. For individuals with coexisting illnesses, medication could comprise of anti-anxiety medication in conjunction with stimulants. Effective cure for depression will happen only when the medicines are taken together.

# Chapter 8

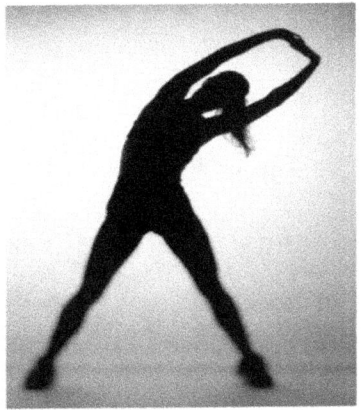

## LIVING WITH DEPRESSION

Living with depression is a lot easier when you have planed

your day.  The best things you can do to overcome a complete

depression cure are:

a)  Take your medicine regularly.

b)  Join self-help groups.

c)  Exercise

d)  Be conscious of your surroundings.

e)  Share your problem.

# Exercises and Self-Help Groups For Depression

The last thing a person wants to do when he or she is depressed is to exercise or mix with people. Depression consumes your inner emotions and feelings. You have the feeling that everything happening around you is 'bad'. Closing your eyes and going to sleep will only give you temporary relief. It will not change unless you do something positive to overcome your depression and have complete depression cure.

a) **Raise up your metabolic rate**: Do small exercises. Raise your hands or swing them around. Be sure to repeat this action when you can throughout the day. You will feel energized and motivated through this one simple step.

b) **Keep notes:** When you write down your feelings – write the darkest ones first – you gain a 'friend'. You are able to relate to something that is not negative. For certain, it may seem 'bad' to you at some point, but then it happens to all of us. Not every one of us is a Shakespeare!

When you share your problem, it will be surprisingly easy to overcome. Writing things down helps you analyze them better and make corrections. It helps you understand what the tough decisions are. and why they are so tough. Once you identify your problems areas, you can discuss them with people you know to find a solution. Your doctor or therapist is the best person to help you.

**Eating nutritious food is vital**. The reason is obvious. When you have dark emotions your metabolism goes into overdrive to compensate for the huge amount of energy required. When this happen include good fats. and foods with phytochemicals that will help overcome loose radicals in our body. Some examples of these foods are:

1) Oysters
2) Wild Salmon
3) Walnuts

4) Chocolates

5) Yam

6) Nuts

Oysters and chocolates belong to the class of aphrodisiac foods. This class of food known as aphrodisiac foods boosts blood flow in the pelvic zones making the person excited. This boost in mood will counterbalance any negative emotions that you feel. Nuts and yams have good fiber content. In addition, omega 3 fatty acids are present in food items like the fish. They help cut down the cholesterol content in the body, and boosts metabolic activities. Overeating carbohydrates such as those found in cereals like wheat or rice and potatoes will make the person slow. That said, carbohydrates remain the best source of energy for the body – but eat it in moderation.

**Food and Lifestyle Changes**

Be aware of what you do. Create a change and check whether your appetite improves. Good health begins with a sound healthy body and a stable conscious mind. That is the first step to overcome depression and have complete depression cure. Begin your trip to consciousness by describing the things around you. Begin with the flower and the grass, and keep repeating how lovely they are day after day. After you have adapted to this change, you are ready for higher and better things. Changing your lifestyle begins when your mind is prepared. And taking your medicine is very essential for all progress.

Your brain has nerve cells that will not communicate like they normally do. Medicines will open up the way for these cells to communicate, and this will stabilize your emotions and moods. When your body does not get its daily nourishment, you can fall back into depression again. Eat your food.

Food gives you the energy needed to complete everyday tasks. To make full use of the energy, you must exercise. Exercise turns the energy into muscles, and the more muscles give strength to the body, you gain better body balance, and you carry lesser weight when you move. Have protein supplements when you begin to really exercise. The body will need the energy and the proteins will assist in muscle growth. When the body structure is strong, one can overcome depression faster.

All of us are depressed some time in our life. The way forward is to overcome our temporary setback and look forward, and act in a positive manner that will help us achieve wonderful things. Remember, if you feel really bad contact your doctor or someone near you – your friend or family member. There is a way to overcome depression and be completely depression free...but you must try. If you know someone who has these symptoms, help them by taking them to a physician or psychiatrist. Depression does not want your sympathy, it wants your action.

# **Conclusion**

Thank you again for choosing this book!

I hope this book was able to help you to overcome your depression.

The next step is to just do it!

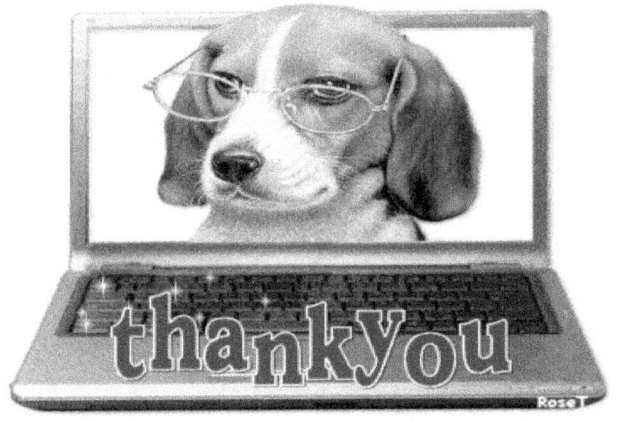

Finally, if you enjoyed this book would you be kind enough to leave a review for this book on Amazon? It'd be greatly appreciated!

Thank you and good luck!

# Preview of "SOCIAL ANXIETY: How to Slay Social Anxiety"

## Chapter 1

### SOCIAL ANXIETY

A definition of social anxiety disorder was provided in 1994 by the American Psychiatric Association in the diagnostic and Statistic Manual of Mental Disorders, defines social anxiety disorder as "a mark and persistent fear of one or more social or performance situations in which the person is exposed to unfamiliar people or possible scrutiny by others.

The person fears that he or she will act in a way (or show anxiety symptoms) that will be humiliating or embarrassing. This means that the heart of social anxiety disorder is anxiety due to concern about what others might think of you.

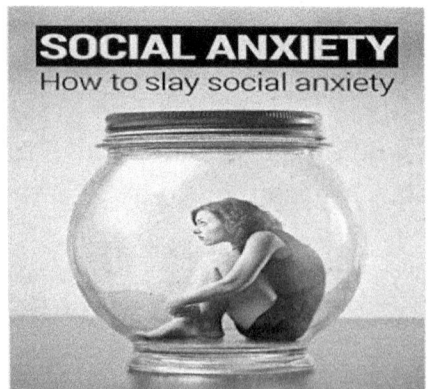

check out the rest of (SOCIAL ANXIETY: How to slay social anxiety) on Amazon.

# Check Out My Other Books

Below you'll find some of my other popular books that are popular on Amazon and Kindle as well. Alternatively, you can visit my author page on Amazon to see other work done by me.

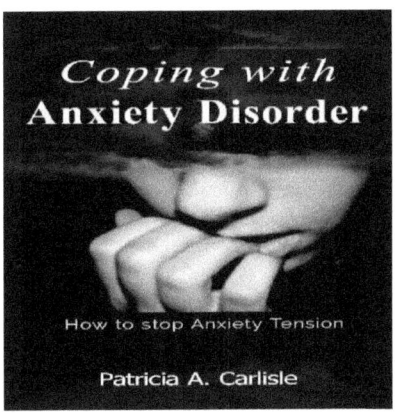

**COPING WITH ANXIETY DISORDER. HOW TO STOP ANXIETY TENSION.**

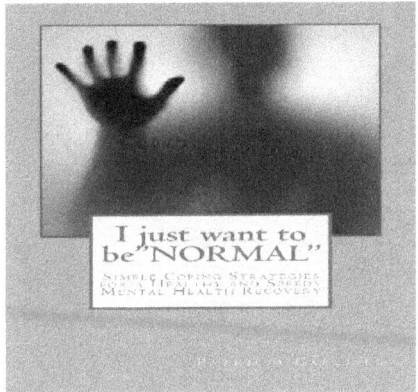

**I JUST WANT TO BE "NORMAL" SIMPLE COPING STRATEGIES FOR A HEALTH A SPEEDY MENTAL HEALTH RECOVERY.**

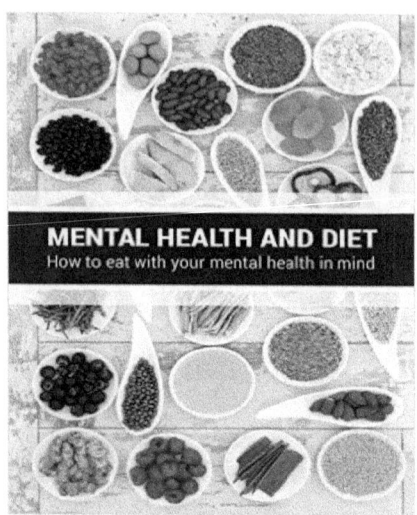

**Mental Health and diet: How to eat with your mental health in mind.**

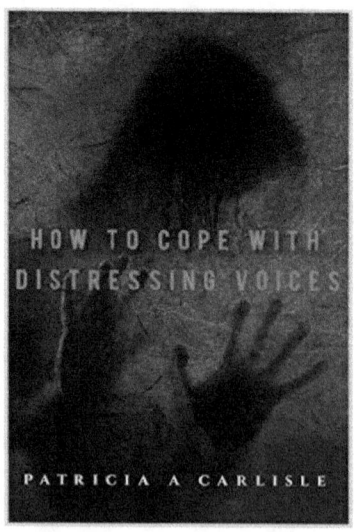

**How to cope with distressing voices.**

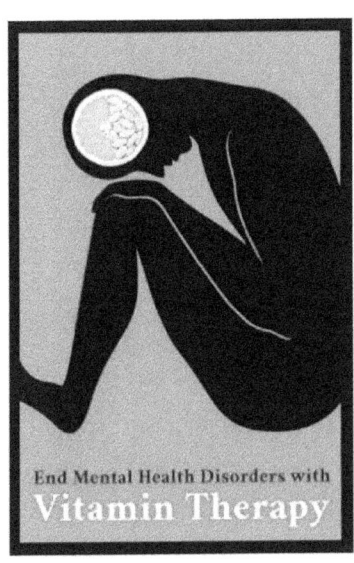

End Mental Health Disorders with Vitamin Therapy.

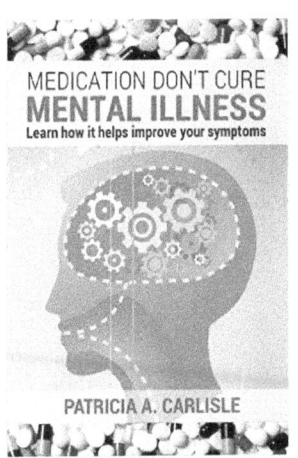

**MEDICATION DON'T CURE MENTAL ILLNESS:**
Learn how it helps improve your symptoms.

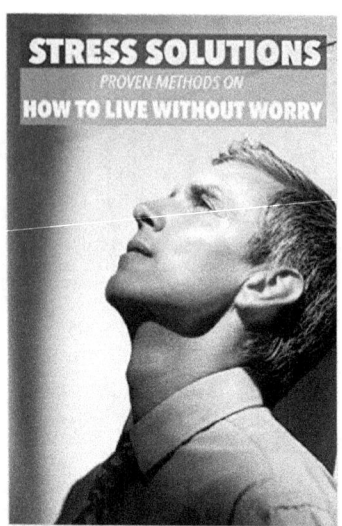

**STRESS SOLUTIONS: Proven methods on how to live without worry.**

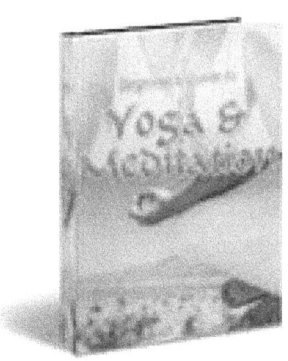

# NOTES

# NOTE

# NOTE

# NOTES